Go Keto with Casey's
12-month record Book

Journal. Log.
Your Diary of Change

Many of us make fresh starts. Often. Like, on a regular basis. Logic tells us that one shouldn't require fresh starts over and over again. And yet …

It is my hope that this little book will help get things on track and keep them there, that the practice of incorporating good habits and shedding those that aren't very good, will result in a fresh start that grows into seasoned permanence.

Fill this journal with words, images, doodles … whatever inspires. By the time you've gotten to the last pages, your life may be altogether different than that reflected in the first pages. Time will tell. And time will pass whether we make changes or not, so we might as well do so, right?

Let the metamorphosis begin!

∞

This is a record of my life as I change it.

The dates covered here are:

_____ *to* _____

Change is made incrementally. One moment, one decision, one hour, one day at a time.

We have more power and are stronger than we think.

- Casey

My big, audacious goal

To Lose 60 lbs
& Gain A Healthy Lifestyle

My personal mission statement

Leaning on Gods strength to help me
Through this journey to a new
Healthy lifestyle.

My plan

The way to get started is to quit talking and begin doing.

- Walt Disney

the month of *Sept* 2024
Oct 2024

MON	TUES	WED	THUR	FRI	SAT	SUN

This month I will: _____

_____

_____

This month I achieved: _____

My words of the month are:

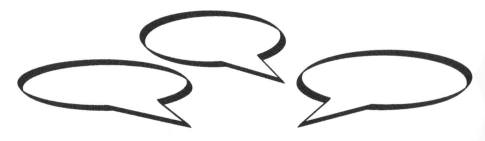

the week of _____

ACHIEVEMENTS

habit tracker

(ADD NEW OR GIVE UP OLD)

M	T	W	T	F	S	S
◯	◯	◯	◯	◯	◯	◯
◯	◯	◯	◯	◯	◯	◯
◯	◯	◯	◯	◯	◯	◯
◯	◯	◯	◯	◯	◯	◯
◯	◯	◯	◯	◯	◯	◯
◯	◯	◯	◯	◯	◯	◯
◯	◯	◯	◯	◯	◯	◯

THOUGHTS, RANDOM & OTHERWISE

the week of _____

ASPIRATIONS   ACHIEVEMENTS

habit tracker

(ADD NEW OR GIVE UP OLD)   **M T W T F S S**

_____   ○ ○ ○ ○ ○ ○ ○

_____   ○ ○ ○ ○ ○ ○ ○

_____   ○ ○ ○ ○ ○ ○ ○

_____   ○ ○ ○ ○ ○ ○ ○

_____   ○ ○ ○ ○ ○ ○ ○

_____   ○ ○ ○ ○ ○ ○ ○

_____   ○ ○ ○ ○ ○ ○ ○

THOUGHTS, RANDOM & OTHERWISE

....
....
....
....
....
....
....
....
....
....

the week of _____

ASPIRATIONS

ACHIEVEMENTS

habit tracker

(ADD NEW OR GIVE UP OLD)

	M	T	W	T	F	S	S
_____	○	○	○	○	○	○	○
_____	○	○	○	○	○	○	○
_____	○	○	○	○	○	○	○
_____	○	○	○	○	○	○	○
_____	○	○	○	○	○	○	○
_____	○	○	○	○	○	○	○
_____	○	○	○	○	○	○	○

THOUGHTS, RANDOM & OTHERWISE

the week of _____

ASPIRATIONS

ACHIEVEMENTS

habit tracker

(ADD NEW OR GIVE UP OLD)

| M | T | W | T | F | S | S |

○ ○ ○ ○ ○ ○ ○

○ ○ ○ ○ ○ ○ ○

○ ○ ○ ○ ○ ○ ○

○ ○ ○ ○ ○ ○ ○

○ ○ ○ ○ ○ ○ ○

○ ○ ○ ○ ○ ○ ○

○ ○ ○ ○ ○ ○ ○

THOUGHTS, RANDOM & OTHERWISE

the week of _____

ASPIRATIONS

ACHIEVEMENTS

habit tracker

(ADD NEW OR GIVE UP OLD)

M	T	W	T	F	S	S
◯	◯	◯	◯	◯	◯	◯
◯	◯	◯	◯	◯	◯	◯
◯	◯	◯	◯	◯	◯	◯
◯	◯	◯	◯	◯	◯	◯
◯	◯	◯	◯	◯	◯	◯
◯	◯	◯	◯	◯	◯	◯
◯	◯	◯	◯	◯	◯	◯

THOUGHTS, RANDOM & OTHERWISE

the month of _____

	HAPPY	"MEH"	TIRED	ANGRY	SAD

1	😊	😐	😑	😠	😢
2	😊	😐	😑	😠	😢
3	😊	😐	😑	😠	😢
4	😊	😐	😑	😠	😢
5	😊	😐	😑	😠	😢
6	😊	😐	😑	😠	😢
7	😊	😐	😑	😠	😢
8	😊	😐	😑	😠	😢
9	😊	😐	😑	😠	😢
10	😊	😐	😑	😠	😢
11	😊	😐	😑	😠	😢
12	😊	😐	😑	😠	😢
13	😊	😐	😑	😠	😢
14	😊	😐	😑	😠	😢
15	😊	😐	😑	😠	😢
16	😊	😐	😑	😠	😢
17	😊	😐	😑	😠	😢
18	😊	😐	😑	😠	😢
19	😊	😐	😑	😠	😢
20	😊	😐	😑	😠	😢
21	😊	😐	😑	😠	😢
22	😊	😐	😑	😠	😢
23	😊	😐	😑	😠	😢
24	😊	😐	😑	😠	😢
25	😊	😐	😑	😠	😢
26	😊	😐	😑	😠	😢
27	😊	😐	😑	😠	😢
28	😊	😐	😑	😠	😢
29	😊	😐	😑	😠	😢
30	😊	😐	😑	😠	😢
31	😊	😐	😑	😠	😢

Inspiration. Motivation. Determination.

A PLACE FOR DOODLES, PHOTOS, STICKERS & WHATEVER MOVES YOU

A PLACE FOR DOODLES, PHOTOS, STICKERS & WHATEVER MOVES YOU

DO OR DO NOT. THERE IS NO TRY.

-Yoda

the month of _____

MON	TUES	WED	THUR	FRI	SAT	SUN

THIS MONTH I WILL: _____
_____
_____

THIS MONTH I ACHIEVED: _____

MY WORDS OF THE MONTH ARE:

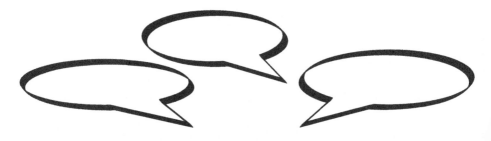

the week of _____

ASPIRATIONS

ACHIEVEMENTS

habit tracker

(ADD NEW OR GIVE UP OLD)

M	T	W	T	F	S	S

_____ ◯ ◯ ◯ ◯ ◯ ◯ ◯

_____ ◯ ◯ ◯ ◯ ◯ ◯ ◯

_____ ◯ ◯ ◯ ◯ ◯ ◯ ◯

_____ ◯ ◯ ◯ ◯ ◯ ◯ ◯

_____ ◯ ◯ ◯ ◯ ◯ ◯ ◯

_____ ◯ ◯ ◯ ◯ ◯ ◯ ◯

_____ ◯ ◯ ◯ ◯ ◯ ◯ ◯

THOUGHTS, RANDOM & OTHERWISE

....
....
....
....
....
....
....
....
....
....
....

the week of _____

ASPIRATIONS

ACHIEVEMENTS

habit tracker

(ADD NEW OR GIVE UP OLD)

M	T	W	T	F	S	S
◯	◯	◯	◯	◯	◯	◯
◯	◯	◯	◯	◯	◯	◯
◯	◯	◯	◯	◯	◯	◯
◯	◯	◯	◯	◯	◯	◯
◯	◯	◯	◯	◯	◯	◯
◯	◯	◯	◯	◯	◯	◯
◯	◯	◯	◯	◯	◯	◯

THOUGHTS, RANDOM & OTHERWISE

....
....
....
....
....
....
....
....
....
....

the week of _____

habit tracker

(ADD NEW OR GIVE UP OLD)

M	T	W	T	F	S	S
◯	◯	◯	◯	◯	◯	◯
◯	◯	◯	◯	◯	◯	◯
◯	◯	◯	◯	◯	◯	◯
◯	◯	◯	◯	◯	◯	◯
◯	◯	◯	◯	◯	◯	◯
◯	◯	◯	◯	◯	◯	◯
◯	◯	◯	◯	◯	◯	◯

THOUGHTS, RANDOM & OTHERWISE

the week of _____

ASPIRATIONS   ACHIEVEMENTS

habit tracker

(ADD NEW OR GIVE UP OLD)   **M** **T** **W** **T** **F** **S** **S**

_____ ○ ○ ○ ○ ○ ○ ○

_____ ○ ○ ○ ○ ○ ○ ○

_____ ○ ○ ○ ○ ○ ○ ○

_____ ○ ○ ○ ○ ○ ○ ○

_____ ○ ○ ○ ○ ○ ○ ○

_____ ○ ○ ○ ○ ○ ○ ○

_____ ○ ○ ○ ○ ○ ○ ○

THOUGHTS, RANDOM & OTHERWISE

....

....

....

....

....

....

....

....

....

the week of _____

habit tracker

(ADD NEW OR GIVE UP OLD)

	M	T	W	T	F	S	S
_____	○	○	○	○	○	○	○
_____	○	○	○	○	○	○	○
_____	○	○	○	○	○	○	○
_____	○	○	○	○	○	○	○
_____	○	○	○	○	○	○	○
_____	○	○	○	○	○	○	○
_____	○	○	○	○	○	○	○

THOUGHTS, RANDOM & OTHERWISE

the month of _____

| | HAPPY | "MEH" | TIRED | ANGRY | SAD |

1
3
5
7
9
11
13
15
17
19
21
23
25
27
29
31

2
4
6
8
10
12
14
16
18
20
22
24
26
28
30

INSPIRATION. MOTIVATION. DETERMINATION.

A PLACE FOR DOODLES, PHOTOS, STICKERS & WHATEVER MOVES YOU

A PLACE FOR DOODLES, PHOTOS, STICKERS & WHATEVER MOVES YOU

It is never too late
to be what you
might have been

- George Eliot

the month of _____

MON	TUES	WED	THUR	FRI	SAT	SUN

THIS MONTH I WILL: _____
_____

THIS MONTH I ACHIEVED: _____

MY WORDS OF THE MONTH ARE:

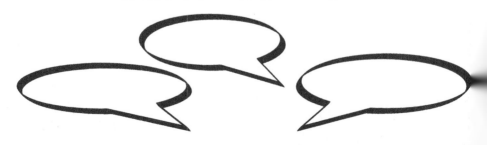

the week of _____

ASPIRATIONS

ACHIEVEMENTS

habit tracker

(ADD NEW OR GIVE UP OLD)   **M T W T F S S**

THOUGHTS, RANDOM & OTHERWISE

the week of _____

ASPIRATIONS | ACHIEVEMENTS

habit tracker

(ADD NEW OR GIVE UP OLD) **M T W T F S S**

_____

_____

_____

_____

_____

_____

_____

THOUGHTS, RANDOM & OTHERWISE

....
....
....
....
....
....
....
....
....
....

the week of _____

ASPIRATIONS

ACHIEVEMENTS

habit tracker

(ADD NEW OR GIVE UP OLD)

M	T	W	T	F	S	S
◯	◯	◯	◯	◯	◯	◯
◯	◯	◯	◯	◯	◯	◯
◯	◯	◯	◯	◯	◯	◯
◯	◯	◯	◯	◯	◯	◯
◯	◯	◯	◯	◯	◯	◯
◯	◯	◯	◯	◯	◯	◯
◯	◯	◯	◯	◯	◯	◯

THOUGHTS, RANDOM & OTHERWISE

the week of _____

ASPIRATIONS

ACHIEVEMENTS

habit tracker

(ADD NEW OR GIVE UP OLD)

M	T	W	T	F	S	S
○	○	○	○	○	○	○
○	○	○	○	○	○	○
○	○	○	○	○	○	○
○	○	○	○	○	○	○
○	○	○	○	○	○	○
○	○	○	○	○	○	○
○	○	○	○	○	○	○

THOUGHTS, RANDOM & OTHERWISE

the week of _____

ASPIRATIONS

ACHIEVEMENTS

habit tracker

(ADD NEW OR GIVE UP OLD)

M	T	W	T	F	S	S

_____

_____

_____

_____

_____

_____

THOUGHTS, RANDOM & OTHERWISE

the month of _____

	HAPPY	"MEH"	TIRED	ANGRY	SAD

1						2					
3						4					
5						6					
7						8					
9						10					
11						12					
13						14					
15						16					
17						18					
19						20					
21						22					
23						24					
25						26					
27						28					
29						30					
31											

INSPIRATION. MOTIVATION. DETERMINATION.

A PLACE FOR DOODLES, PHOTOS, STICKERS & WHATEVER MOVES YOU

A PLACE FOR DOODLES, PHOTOS, STICKERS & WHATEVER MOVES YOU

Be yourself: everyone else is already taken.

- Oscar Wilde (*attributed to*)

the month of _____

MON	TUES	WED	THUR	FRI	SAT	SUN

THIS MONTH I WILL: _____
_____

THIS MONTH I ACHIEVED: _____

MY WORDS OF THE MONTH ARE:

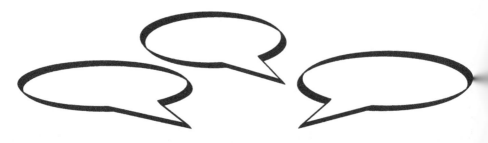

the week of _____

ASPIRATIONS   ACHIEVEMENTS

habit tracker

(ADD NEW OR GIVE UP OLD)   **M** **T** **W** **T** **F** **S** **S**

_____ ○ ○ ○ ○ ○ ○ ○

_____ ○ ○ ○ ○ ○ ○ ○

_____ ○ ○ ○ ○ ○ ○ ○

_____ ○ ○ ○ ○ ○ ○ ○

_____ ○ ○ ○ ○ ○ ○ ○

_____ ○ ○ ○ ○ ○ ○ ○

_____ ○ ○ ○ ○ ○ ○ ○

THOUGHTS, RANDOM & OTHERWISE

....
....
....
....
....
....
....
....
....
....
....

ASPIRATIONS

ACHIEVEMENTS

habit tracker

(ADD NEW OR GIVE UP OLD)

M	T	W	T	F	S	S
○	○	○	○	○	○	○
○	○	○	○	○	○	○
○	○	○	○	○	○	○
○	○	○	○	○	○	○
○	○	○	○	○	○	○
○	○	○	○	○	○	○
○	○	○	○	○	○	○

THOUGHTS, RANDOM & OTHERWISE

the week of _____

ASPIRATIONS

ACHIEVEMENTS

habit tracker

(ADD NEW OR GIVE UP OLD)

M	T	W	T	F	S	S
◯	◯	◯	◯	◯	◯	◯
◯	◯	◯	◯	◯	◯	◯
◯	◯	◯	◯	◯	◯	◯
◯	◯	◯	◯	◯	◯	◯
◯	◯	◯	◯	◯	◯	◯
◯	◯	◯	◯	◯	◯	◯
◯	◯	◯	◯	◯	◯	◯

THOUGHTS, RANDOM & OTHERWISE

the week of _____

ASPIRATIONS   ACHIEVEMENTS

habit tracker

(ADD NEW OR GIVE UP OLD)   **M T W T F S S**

_____ ○ ○ ○ ○ ○ ○ ○

_____ ○ ○ ○ ○ ○ ○ ○

_____ ○ ○ ○ ○ ○ ○ ○

_____ ○ ○ ○ ○ ○ ○ ○

_____ ○ ○ ○ ○ ○ ○ ○

_____ ○ ○ ○ ○ ○ ○ ○

_____ ○ ○ ○ ○ ○ ○ ○

THOUGHTS, RANDOM & OTHERWISE

....
....
....
....
....
....
....
....
....
....
....

the week of _____

ASPIRATIONS

ACHIEVEMENTS

habit tracker

(ADD NEW OR GIVE UP OLD)

M	T	W	T	F	S	S
◯	◯	◯	◯	◯	◯	◯
◯	◯	◯	◯	◯	◯	◯
◯	◯	◯	◯	◯	◯	◯
◯	◯	◯	◯	◯	◯	◯
◯	◯	◯	◯	◯	◯	◯
◯	◯	◯	◯	◯	◯	◯
◯	◯	◯	◯	◯	◯	◯

THOUGHTS, RANDOM & OTHERWISE

the month of _____

	HAPPY	"MEH"	TIRED	ANGRY	SAD

1
2
3
4
5
6
7
8
9
10
11
12
13
14
15
16
17
18
19
20
21
22
23
24
25
26
27
28
29
30
31

INSPIRATION. MOTIVATION. DETERMINATION.

A PLACE FOR DOODLES, PHOTOS, STICKERS & WHATEVER MOVES YOU

A PLACE FOR DOODLES, PHOTOS, STICKERS & WHATEVER MOVES YOU

If a problem has a solution, there is no need to worry.
If a problem has no solution, worry is of no use.

- His Holiness the 14th Dalai Lama

the month of _____

MON	TUES	WED	THUR	FRI	SAT	SUN

THIS MONTH I WILL: _____

_____

_____

THIS MONTH I ACHIEVED: _____

MY WORDS OF THE MONTH ARE:

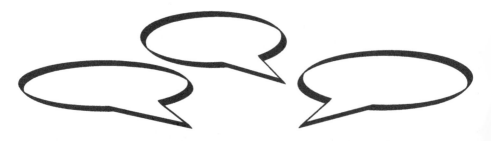

the week of _____

ASPIRATIONS

ACHIEVEMENTS

habit tracker

(ADD NEW OR GIVE UP OLD)

M	T	W	T	F	S	S
○	○	○	○	○	○	○
○	○	○	○	○	○	○
○	○	○	○	○	○	○
○	○	○	○	○	○	○
○	○	○	○	○	○	○
○	○	○	○	○	○	○
○	○	○	○	○	○	○

THOUGHTS, RANDOM & OTHERWISE

the week of _____

habit tracker

(ADD NEW OR GIVE UP OLD)

M	T	W	T	F	S	S
◯	◯	◯	◯	◯	◯	◯
◯	◯	◯	◯	◯	◯	◯
◯	◯	◯	◯	◯	◯	◯
◯	◯	◯	◯	◯	◯	◯
◯	◯	◯	◯	◯	◯	◯
◯	◯	◯	◯	◯	◯	◯
◯	◯	◯	◯	◯	◯	◯

THOUGHTS, RANDOM & OTHERWISE

the week of _____

ASPIRATIONS

ACHIEVEMENTS

habit tracker

(ADD NEW OR GIVE UP OLD)

M	T	W	T	F	S	S
○	○	○	○	○	○	○
○	○	○	○	○	○	○
○	○	○	○	○	○	○
○	○	○	○	○	○	○
○	○	○	○	○	○	○
○	○	○	○	○	○	○
○	○	○	○	○	○	○

THOUGHTS, RANDOM & OTHERWISE

the week of _____

ASPIRATIONS

ACHIEVEMENTS

habit tracker

(ADD NEW OR GIVE UP OLD)

M	T	W	T	F	S	S
◯	◯	◯	◯	◯	◯	◯
◯	◯	◯	◯	◯	◯	◯
◯	◯	◯	◯	◯	◯	◯
◯	◯	◯	◯	◯	◯	◯
◯	◯	◯	◯	◯	◯	◯
◯	◯	◯	◯	◯	◯	◯
◯	◯	◯	◯	◯	◯	◯

THOUGHTS, RANDOM & OTHERWISE

the week of _____

ASPIRATIONS

ACHIEVEMENTS

habit tracker

(ADD NEW OR GIVE UP OLD)

M	T	W	T	F	S	S
○	○	○	○	○	○	○
○	○	○	○	○	○	○
○	○	○	○	○	○	○
○	○	○	○	○	○	○
○	○	○	○	○	○	○
○	○	○	○	○	○	○
○	○	○	○	○	○	○

THOUGHTS, RANDOM & OTHERWISE

the month of _____

| | HAPPY | "MEH" | TIRED | ANGRY | SAD |

1 😀 😊 😑 😠 😢   2 😀 😊 😑 😠 😢

3 😀 😊 😑 😠 😢   4 😀 😊 😑 😠 😢

5 😀 😊 😑 😠 😢   6 😀 😊 😑 😠 😢

7 😀 😊 😑 😠 😢   8 😀 😊 😑 😠 😢

9 😀 😊 😑 😠 😢   10 😀 😊 😑 😠 😢

11 😀 😊 😑 😠 😢   12 😀 😊 😑 😠 😢

13 😀 😊 😑 😠 😢   14 😀 😊 😑 😠 😢

15 😀 😊 😑 😠 😢   16 😀 😊 😑 😠 😢

17 😀 😊 😑 😠 😢   18 😀 😊 😑 😠 😢

19 😀 😊 😑 😠 😢   20 😀 😊 😑 😠 😢

21 😀 😊 😑 😠 😢   22 😀 😊 😑 😠 😢

23 😀 😊 😑 😠 😢   24 😀 😊 😑 😠 😢

25 😀 😊 😑 😠 😢   26 😀 😊 😑 😠 😢

27 😀 😊 😑 😠 😢   28 😀 😊 😑 😠 😢

29 😀 😊 😑 😠 😢   30 😀 😊 😑 😠 😢

31 😀 😊 😑 😠 😢

INSPIRATION. MOTIVATION. DETERMINATION.

A PLACE FOR DOODLES, PHOTOS, STICKERS & WHATEVER MOVES YOU

A PLACE FOR DOODLES, PHOTOS, STICKERS & WHATEVER MOVES YOU

Keto is simple, which is not to say it is easy.

But just because it isn't easy doesn't mean you can't do it.

-Casey

the month of _____

MON	TUES	WED	THUR	FRI	SAT	SUN

THIS MONTH I WILL: _____

_____

_____

THIS MONTH I ACHIEVED: _____

MY WORDS OF THE MONTH ARE:

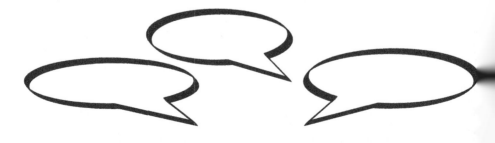

the week of

ASPIRATIONS

ACHIEVEMENTS

habit tracker

(ADD NEW OR GIVE UP OLD)

M	T	W	T	F	S	S

THOUGHTS, RANDOM & OTHERWISE

the week of _____

ASPIRATIONS

ACHIEVEMENTS

habit tracker

(ADD NEW OR GIVE UP OLD)

M	T	W	T	F	S	S
◯	◯	◯	◯	◯	◯	◯
◯	◯	◯	◯	◯	◯	◯
◯	◯	◯	◯	◯	◯	◯
◯	◯	◯	◯	◯	◯	◯
◯	◯	◯	◯	◯	◯	◯
◯	◯	◯	◯	◯	◯	◯
◯	◯	◯	◯	◯	◯	◯

THOUGHTS, RANDOM & OTHERWISE

the week of _____

ASPIRATIONS

ACHIEVEMENTS

habit tracker

(ADD NEW OR GIVE UP OLD)

M	T	W	T	F	S	S
◯	◯	◯	◯	◯	◯	◯
◯	◯	◯	◯	◯	◯	◯
◯	◯	◯	◯	◯	◯	◯
◯	◯	◯	◯	◯	◯	◯
◯	◯	◯	◯	◯	◯	◯
◯	◯	◯	◯	◯	◯	◯
◯	◯	◯	◯	◯	◯	◯

THOUGHTS, RANDOM & OTHERWISE

the week of _____

habit tracker

(ADD NEW OR GIVE UP OLD)

M	T	W	T	F	S	S
◯	◯	◯	◯	◯	◯	◯
◯	◯	◯	◯	◯	◯	◯
◯	◯	◯	◯	◯	◯	◯
◯	◯	◯	◯	◯	◯	◯
◯	◯	◯	◯	◯	◯	◯
◯	◯	◯	◯	◯	◯	◯
◯	◯	◯	◯	◯	◯	◯

THOUGHTS, RANDOM & OTHERWISE

the week of _____

ASPIRATIONS

ACHIEVEMENTS

habit tracker

(ADD NEW OR GIVE UP OLD)

M	T	W	T	F	S	S

_____

_____

_____

_____

_____

THOUGHTS, RANDOM & OTHERWISE

the month of

_____

| HAPPY | "MEH" | TIRED | ANGRY | SAD |

1

2

3

4

5

6

7

8

9

10

11

12

13

14

15

16

17

18

19

20

21

22

23

24

25

26

27

28

29

30

31

INSPIRATION. MOTIVATION. DETERMINATION.

A PLACE FOR DOODLES, PHOTOS, STICKERS & WHATEVER MOVES YOU

A PLACE FOR DOODLES, PHOTOS, STICKERS & WHATEVER MOVES YOU

When you
reach the end
of your rope,
tie a knot in it
and hang on.

- Franklin D. Roosevelt

the month of _____

MON	TUES	WED	THUR	FRI	SAT	SUN

THIS MONTH I WILL: _____
_____
_____

THIS MONTH I ACHIEVED: _____

MY WORDS OF THE MONTH ARE:

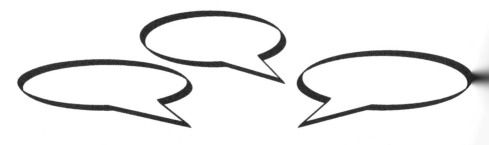

the week of _____

habit tracker

(ADD NEW OR GIVE UP OLD)

M	T	W	T	F	S	S
○	○	○	○	○	○	○
○	○	○	○	○	○	○
○	○	○	○	○	○	○
○	○	○	○	○	○	○
○	○	○	○	○	○	○
○	○	○	○	○	○	○
○	○	○	○	○	○	○

THOUGHTS, RANDOM & OTHERWISE

the week of _____

ASPIRATIONS

ACHIEVEMENTS

habit tracker

(ADD NEW OR GIVE UP OLD)

M	T	W	T	F	S	S

_____

_____

_____

_____

_____

_____

_____

THOUGHTS, RANDOM & OTHERWISE

the week of _____

ASPIRATIONS

ACHIEVEMENTS

habit tracker

(ADD NEW OR GIVE UP OLD)

M	T	W	T	F	S	S
○	○	○	○	○	○	○
○	○	○	○	○	○	○
○	○	○	○	○	○	○
○	○	○	○	○	○	○
○	○	○	○	○	○	○
○	○	○	○	○	○	○
○	○	○	○	○	○	○

THOUGHTS, RANDOM & OTHERWISE

the week of _____

ASPIRATIONS | ACHIEVEMENTS

habit tracker

(ADD NEW OR GIVE UP OLD)

M	T	W	T	F	S	S

_____

_____

_____

_____

_____

_____

_____

THOUGHTS, RANDOM & OTHERWISE

....
....
....
....
....
....
....
....
....
....

the week of _____

ASPIRATIONS

ACHIEVEMENTS

habit tracker

(ADD NEW OR GIVE UP OLD)

M	T	W	T	F	S	S

_____ ○ ○ ○ ○ ○ ○ ○

_____ ○ ○ ○ ○ ○ ○ ○

_____ ○ ○ ○ ○ ○ ○ ○

_____ ○ ○ ○ ○ ○ ○ ○

_____ ○ ○ ○ ○ ○ ○ ○

_____ ○ ○ ○ ○ ○ ○ ○

_____ ○ ○ ○ ○ ○ ○ ○

THOUGHTS, RANDOM & OTHERWISE

	HAPPY	"MEH"	TIRED	ANGRY	SAD

1   😀 😐 😑 😠 😞   2   😀 😐 😑 😠 😞

3   😀 😐 😑 😠 😞   4   😀 😐 😑 😠 😞

5   😀 😐 😑 😠 😞   6   😀 😐 😑 😠 😞

7   😀 😐 😑 😠 😞   8   😀 😐 😑 😠 😞

9   😀 😐 😑 😠 😞   10   😀 😐 😑 😠 😞

11   😀 😐 😑 😠 😞   12   😀 😐 😑 😠 😞

13   😀 😐 😑 😠 😞   14   😀 😐 😑 😠 😞

15   😀 😐 😑 😠 😞   16   😀 😐 😑 😠 😞

17   😀 😐 😑 😠 😞   18   😀 😐 😑 😠 😞

19   😀 😐 😑 😠 😞   20   😀 😐 😑 😠 😞

21   😀 😐 😑 😠 😞   22   😀 😐 😑 😠 😞

23   😀 😐 😑 😠 😞   24   😀 😐 😑 😠 😞

25   😀 😐 😑 😠 😞   26   😀 😐 😑 😠 😞

27   😀 😐 😑 😠 😞   28   😀 😐 😑 😠 😞

29   😀 😐 😑 😠 😞   30   😀 😐 😑 😠 😞

31   😀 😐 😑 😠 😞

INSPIRATION. MOTIVATION. DETERMINATION.

A PLACE FOR DOODLES, PHOTOS, STICKERS & WHATEVER MOVES YOU

A PLACE FOR DOODLES, PHOTOS, STICKERS & WHATEVER MOVES YOU

You only live once,
but if you do it right,
once is enough.

- Mae West

the month of _____

MON	TUES	WED	THUR	FRI	SAT	SUN

THIS MONTH I WILL: _____
_____

THIS MONTH I ACHIEVED: _____

MY WORDS OF THE MONTH ARE:

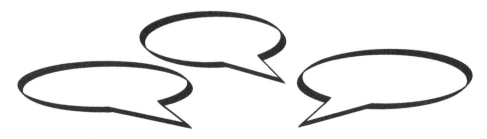

the week of _____

ASPIRATIONS

ACHIEVEMENTS

habit tracker

(ADD NEW OR GIVE UP OLD)

M	T	W	T	F	S	S
◯	◯	◯	◯	◯	◯	◯
◯	◯	◯	◯	◯	◯	◯
◯	◯	◯	◯	◯	◯	◯
◯	◯	◯	◯	◯	◯	◯
◯	◯	◯	◯	◯	◯	◯
◯	◯	◯	◯	◯	◯	◯
◯	◯	◯	◯	◯	◯	◯

THOUGHTS, RANDOM & OTHERWISE

the week of _____

ASPIRATIONS   ACHIEVEMENTS

habit tracker

(ADD NEW OR GIVE UP OLD)   **M   T   W   T   F   S   S**

THOUGHTS, RANDOM & OTHERWISE

the week of _____

habit tracker

(ADD NEW OR GIVE UP OLD)

M	T	W	T	F	S	S
◯	◯	◯	◯	◯	◯	◯
◯	◯	◯	◯	◯	◯	◯
◯	◯	◯	◯	◯	◯	◯
◯	◯	◯	◯	◯	◯	◯
◯	◯	◯	◯	◯	◯	◯
◯	◯	◯	◯	◯	◯	◯
◯	◯	◯	◯	◯	◯	◯

THOUGHTS, RANDOM & OTHERWISE

the week of

ASPIRATIONS

ACHIEVEMENTS

habit tracker

(ADD NEW OR GIVE UP OLD)

M	T	W	T	F	S	S
○	○	○	○	○	○	○
○	○	○	○	○	○	○
○	○	○	○	○	○	○
○	○	○	○	○	○	○
○	○	○	○	○	○	○
○	○	○	○	○	○	○
○	○	○	○	○	○	○

THOUGHTS, RANDOM & OTHERWISE

the week of _____

ASPIRATIONS

ACHIEVEMENTS

habit tracker

(ADD NEW OR GIVE UP OLD)

M	T	W	T	F	S	S
○	○	○	○	○	○	○
○	○	○	○	○	○	○
○	○	○	○	○	○	○
○	○	○	○	○	○	○
○	○	○	○	○	○	○
○	○	○	○	○	○	○
○	○	○	○	○	○	○

THOUGHTS, RANDOM & OTHERWISE

the month of _____

	HAPPY	"MEH"	TIRED	ANGRY	SAD

1 😄 😐 😑 😠 😢   2 😄 😐 😑 😠 😢

3 😄 😐 😑 😠 😢   4 😄 😐 😑 😠 😢

5 😄 😐 😑 😠 😢   6 😄 😐 😑 😠 😢

7 😄 😐 😑 😠 😢   8 😄 😐 😑 😠 😢

9 😄 😐 😑 😠 😢   10 😄 😐 😑 😠 😢

11 😄 😐 😑 😠 😢   12 😄 😐 😑 😠 😢

13 😄 😐 😑 😠 😢   14 😄 😐 😑 😠 😢

15 😄 😐 😑 😠 😢   16 😄 😐 😑 😠 😢

17 😄 😐 😑 😠 😢   18 😄 😐 😑 😠 😢

19 😄 😐 😑 😠 😢   20 😄 😐 😑 😠 😢

21 😄 😐 😑 😠 😢   22 😄 😐 😑 😠 😢

23 😄 😐 😑 😠 😢   24 😄 😐 😑 😠 😢

25 😄 😐 😑 😠 😢   26 😄 😐 😑 😠 😢

27 😄 😐 😑 😠 😢   28 😄 😐 😑 😠 😢

29 😄 😐 😑 😠 😢   30 😄 😐 😑 😠 😢

31 😄 😐 😑 😠 😢

INSPIRATION. MOTIVATION. DETERMINATION.

A PLACE FOR DOODLES, PHOTOS, STICKERS & WHATEVER MOVES YOU

A PLACE FOR DOODLES, PHOTOS, STICKERS & WHATEVER MOVES YOU

Life is really
simple, but we
insist on making it
complicated

- Confucius

the month of _____

MON	TUES	WED	THUR	FRI	SAT	SUN

THIS MONTH I WILL: _____
_____
_____

THIS MONTH I ACHIEVED: _____

MY WORDS OF THE MONTH ARE:

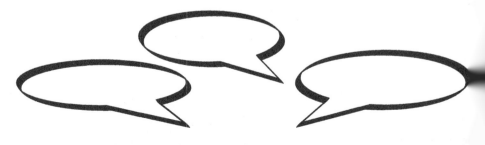

the week of _____

habit tracker

(ADD NEW OR GIVE UP OLD)

M	T	W	T	F	S	S
◯	◯	◯	◯	◯	◯	◯
◯	◯	◯	◯	◯	◯	◯
◯	◯	◯	◯	◯	◯	◯
◯	◯	◯	◯	◯	◯	◯
◯	◯	◯	◯	◯	◯	◯
◯	◯	◯	◯	◯	◯	◯
◯	◯	◯	◯	◯	◯	◯

THOUGHTS, RANDOM & OTHERWISE

the week of _____

ASPIRATIONS

ACHIEVEMENTS

habit tracker

(ADD NEW OR GIVE UP OLD)

M	T	W	T	F	S	S
○	○	○	○	○	○	○
○	○	○	○	○	○	○
○	○	○	○	○	○	○
○	○	○	○	○	○	○
○	○	○	○	○	○	○
○	○	○	○	○	○	○
○	○	○	○	○	○	○

THOUGHTS, RANDOM & OTHERWISE

the week of _____

habit tracker

(ADD NEW OR GIVE UP OLD)

M	T	W	T	F	S	S
◯	◯	◯	◯	◯	◯	◯
◯	◯	◯	◯	◯	◯	◯
◯	◯	◯	◯	◯	◯	◯
◯	◯	◯	◯	◯	◯	◯
◯	◯	◯	◯	◯	◯	◯
◯	◯	◯	◯	◯	◯	◯
◯	◯	◯	◯	◯	◯	◯

THOUGHTS, RANDOM & OTHERWISE

the week of _____

habit tracker

(ADD NEW OR GIVE UP OLD)

M	T	W	T	F	S	S
◯	◯	◯	◯	◯	◯	◯
◯	◯	◯	◯	◯	◯	◯
◯	◯	◯	◯	◯	◯	◯
◯	◯	◯	◯	◯	◯	◯
◯	◯	◯	◯	◯	◯	◯
◯	◯	◯	◯	◯	◯	◯
◯	◯	◯	◯	◯	◯	◯

THOUGHTS, RANDOM & OTHERWISE

the week of _____

habit tracker

(ADD NEW OR GIVE UP OLD)

M	T	W	T	F	S	S
◯	◯	◯	◯	◯	◯	◯
◯	◯	◯	◯	◯	◯	◯
◯	◯	◯	◯	◯	◯	◯
◯	◯	◯	◯	◯	◯	◯
◯	◯	◯	◯	◯	◯	◯
◯	◯	◯	◯	◯	◯	◯
◯	◯	◯	◯	◯	◯	◯

THOUGHTS, RANDOM & OTHERWISE

the month of _____

	HAPPY	"MEH"	TIRED	ANGRY	SAD

1	😊 😐 😑 😠 🙁		2	😊 😐 😑 😠 🙁
3	😊 😐 😑 😠 🙁		4	😊 😐 😑 😠 🙁
5	😊 😐 😑 😠 🙁		6	😊 😐 😑 😠 🙁
7	😊 😐 😑 😠 🙁		8	😊 😐 😑 😠 🙁
9	😊 😐 😑 😠 🙁		10	😊 😐 😑 😠 🙁
11	😊 😐 😑 😠 🙁		12	😊 😐 😑 😠 🙁
13	😊 😐 😑 😠 🙁		14	😊 😐 😑 😠 🙁
15	😊 😐 😑 😠 🙁		16	😊 😐 😑 😠 🙁
17	😊 😐 😑 😠 🙁		18	😊 😐 😑 😠 🙁
19	😊 😐 😑 😠 🙁		20	😊 😐 😑 😠 🙁
21	😊 😐 😑 😠 🙁		22	😊 😐 😑 😠 🙁
23	😊 😐 😑 😠 🙁		24	😊 😐 😑 😠 🙁
25	😊 😐 😑 😠 🙁		26	😊 😐 😑 😠 🙁
27	😊 😐 😑 😠 🙁		28	😊 😐 😑 😠 🙁
29	😊 😐 😑 😠 🙁		30	😊 😐 😑 😠 🙁
31	😊 😐 😑 😠 🙁			

INSPIRATION. MOTIVATION. DETERMINATION.

A PLACE FOR DOODLES, PHOTOS, STICKERS & WHATEVER MOVES YOU

A PLACE FOR DOODLES, PHOTOS, STICKERS & WHATEVER MOVES YOU

You have brains in your head. You have feet in your shoes. You can steer yourself any direction you choose

- Dr. Seuss

the month of _____

MON	TUES	WED	THUR	FRI	SAT	SUN

THIS MONTH I WILL: _____
_____
_____

THIS MONTH I ACHIEVED: _____

MY WORDS OF THE MONTH ARE:

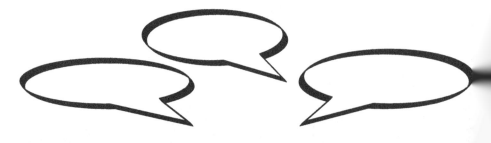

the week of _____

habit tracker

(ADD NEW OR GIVE UP OLD)

M	T	W	T	F	S	S
◯	◯	◯	◯	◯	◯	◯
◯	◯	◯	◯	◯	◯	◯
◯	◯	◯	◯	◯	◯	◯
◯	◯	◯	◯	◯	◯	◯
◯	◯	◯	◯	◯	◯	◯
◯	◯	◯	◯	◯	◯	◯
◯	◯	◯	◯	◯	◯	◯

THOUGHTS, RANDOM & OTHERWISE

the week of _____

ASPIRATIONS   ACHIEVEMENTS

habit tracker

(ADD NEW OR GIVE UP OLD)   **M T W T F S S**

_____

_____

_____

_____

_____

_____

_____

THOUGHTS, RANDOM & OTHERWISE

the week of _____

habit tracker

(ADD NEW OR GIVE UP OLD)

	M	T	W	T	F	S	S
_____	○	○	○	○	○	○	○
_____	○	○	○	○	○	○	○
_____	○	○	○	○	○	○	○
_____	○	○	○	○	○	○	○
_____	○	○	○	○	○	○	○
_____	○	○	○	○	○	○	○
_____	○	○	○	○	○	○	○

THOUGHTS, RANDOM & OTHERWISE

....
....
....
....
....
....
....
....
....
....

the week of _____

ASPIRATIONS

ACHIEVEMENTS

habit tracker

(ADD NEW OR GIVE UP OLD)   **M** **T** **W** **T** **F** **S** **S**

_____ ○ ○ ○ ○ ○ ○ ○

_____ ○ ○ ○ ○ ○ ○ ○

_____ ○ ○ ○ ○ ○ ○ ○

_____ ○ ○ ○ ○ ○ ○ ○

_____ ○ ○ ○ ○ ○ ○ ○

_____ ○ ○ ○ ○ ○ ○ ○

_____ ○ ○ ○ ○ ○ ○ ○

THOUGHTS, RANDOM & OTHERWISE

the week of _____

ASPIRATIONS

ACHIEVEMENTS

habit tracker

(ADD NEW OR GIVE UP OLD)

M	T	W	T	F	S	S
○	○	○	○	○	○	○
○	○	○	○	○	○	○
○	○	○	○	○	○	○
○	○	○	○	○	○	○
○	○	○	○	○	○	○
○	○	○	○	○	○	○
○	○	○	○	○	○	○

THOUGHTS, RANDOM & OTHERWISE

the month of _____

	HAPPY	"MEH"	TIRED	ANGRY	SAD

1	☺ ☺ ☺ ☹ ☹		2	☺ ☺ ☺ ☹ ☹
3	☺ ☺ ☺ ☹ ☹		4	☺ ☺ ☺ ☹ ☹
5	☺ ☺ ☺ ☹ ☹		6	☺ ☺ ☺ ☹ ☹
7	☺ ☺ ☺ ☹ ☹		8	☺ ☺ ☺ ☹ ☹
9	☺ ☺ ☺ ☹ ☹		10	☺ ☺ ☺ ☹ ☹
11	☺ ☺ ☺ ☹ ☹		12	☺ ☺ ☺ ☹ ☹
13	☺ ☺ ☺ ☹ ☹		14	☺ ☺ ☺ ☹ ☹
15	☺ ☺ ☺ ☹ ☹		16	☺ ☺ ☺ ☹ ☹
17	☺ ☺ ☺ ☹ ☹		18	☺ ☺ ☺ ☹ ☹
19	☺ ☺ ☺ ☹ ☹		20	☺ ☺ ☺ ☹ ☹
21	☺ ☺ ☺ ☹ ☹		22	☺ ☺ ☺ ☹ ☹
23	☺ ☺ ☺ ☹ ☹		24	☺ ☺ ☺ ☹ ☹
25	☺ ☺ ☺ ☹ ☹		26	☺ ☺ ☺ ☹ ☹
27	☺ ☺ ☺ ☹ ☹		28	☺ ☺ ☺ ☹ ☹
29	☺ ☺ ☺ ☹ ☹		30	☺ ☺ ☺ ☹ ☹
31	☺ ☺ ☺ ☹ ☹			

INSPIRATION. MOTIVATION. DETERMINATION.

A PLACE FOR DOODLES, PHOTOS, STICKERS & WHATEVER MOVES YOU

A PLACE FOR DOODLES, PHOTOS, STICKERS & WHATEVER MOVES YOU

Many of life's failures are people who did not realize how close they were to success when they gave up.

- Thomas Edison

the month of _____

MON	TUES	WED	THUR	FRI	SAT	SUN

THIS MONTH I WILL: _____

_____

_____

THIS MONTH I ACHIEVED: _____

MY WORDS OF THE MONTH ARE:

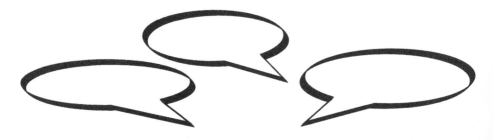

the week of _____

ASPIRATIONS

ACHIEVEMENTS

habit tracker

(ADD NEW OR GIVE UP OLD)

M	T	W	T	F	S	S

_____
_____
_____
_____
_____
_____
_____

THOUGHTS, RANDOM & OTHERWISE

the week of _____

ASPIRATIONS

ACHIEVEMENTS

habit tracker

(ADD NEW OR GIVE UP OLD)

M	T	W	T	F	S	S
○	○	○	○	○	○	○
○	○	○	○	○	○	○
○	○	○	○	○	○	○
○	○	○	○	○	○	○
○	○	○	○	○	○	○
○	○	○	○	○	○	○
○	○	○	○	○	○	○

THOUGHTS, RANDOM & OTHERWISE

the week of _____

habit tracker

(ADD NEW OR GIVE UP OLD)

M	T	W	T	F	S	S
◯	◯	◯	◯	◯	◯	◯
◯	◯	◯	◯	◯	◯	◯
◯	◯	◯	◯	◯	◯	◯
◯	◯	◯	◯	◯	◯	◯
◯	◯	◯	◯	◯	◯	◯
◯	◯	◯	◯	◯	◯	◯
◯	◯	◯	◯	◯	◯	◯

THOUGHTS, RANDOM & OTHERWISE

the week of _____

ASPIRATIONS

ACHIEVEMENTS

habit tracker

(ADD NEW OR GIVE UP OLD)

M	T	W	T	F	S	S
○	○	○	○	○	○	○
○	○	○	○	○	○	○
○	○	○	○	○	○	○
○	○	○	○	○	○	○
○	○	○	○	○	○	○
○	○	○	○	○	○	○
○	○	○	○	○	○	○

THOUGHTS, RANDOM & OTHERWISE

the week of _____

habit tracker

(ADD NEW OR GIVE UP OLD)

	M	T	W	T	F	S	S
_____	○	○	○	○	○	○	○
_____	○	○	○	○	○	○	○
_____	○	○	○	○	○	○	○
_____	○	○	○	○	○	○	○
_____	○	○	○	○	○	○	○
_____	○	○	○	○	○	○	○
_____	○	○	○	○	○	○	○

THOUGHTS, RANDOM & OTHERWISE

the month of _____

	HAPPY	"MEH"	TIRED	ANGRY	SAD

1 😊 😐 😑 😠 😢   2 😊 😐 😑 😠 😢

3 😊 😐 😑 😠 😢   4 😊 😐 😑 😠 😢

5 😊 😐 😑 😠 😢   6 😊 😐 😑 😠 😢

7 😊 😐 😑 😠 😢   8 😊 😐 😑 😠 😢

9 😊 😐 😑 😠 😢   10 😊 😐 😑 😠 😢

11 😊 😐 😑 😠 😢   12 😊 😐 😑 😠 😢

13 😊 😐 😑 😠 😢   14 😊 😐 😑 😠 😢

15 😊 😐 😑 😠 😢   16 😊 😐 😑 😠 😢

17 😊 😐 😑 😠 😢   18 😊 😐 😑 😠 😢

19 😊 😐 😑 😠 😢   20 😊 😐 😑 😠 😢

21 😊 😐 😑 😠 😢   22 😊 😐 😑 😠 😢

23 😊 😐 😑 😠 😢   24 😊 😐 😑 😠 😢

25 😊 😐 😑 😠 😢   26 😊 😐 😑 😠 😢

27 😊 😐 😑 😠 😢   28 😊 😐 😑 😠 😢

29 😊 😐 😑 😠 😢   30 😊 😐 😑 😠 😢

31 😊 😐 😑 😠 😢

Inspiration. Motivation. Determination.

A PLACE FOR DOODLES, PHOTOS, STICKERS & WHATEVER MOVES YOU

A PLACE FOR DOODLES, PHOTOS, STICKERS & WHATEVER MOVES YOU

The sun don't shine on the same dog's ass every day.

- (stolen by) Casey

the month of _____

MON	TUES	WED	THUR	FRI	SAT	SUN

THIS MONTH I WILL: _____
_____
_____

THIS MONTH I ACHIEVED: _____

MY WORDS OF THE MONTH ARE:

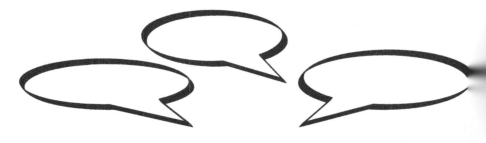

the week of _____

ASPIRATIONS

ACHIEVEMENTS

habit tracker

(ADD NEW OR GIVE UP OLD)

M	T	W	T	F	S	S
◯	◯	◯	◯	◯	◯	◯
◯	◯	◯	◯	◯	◯	◯
◯	◯	◯	◯	◯	◯	◯
◯	◯	◯	◯	◯	◯	◯
◯	◯	◯	◯	◯	◯	◯
◯	◯	◯	◯	◯	◯	◯
◯	◯	◯	◯	◯	◯	◯

THOUGHTS, RANDOM & OTHERWISE

ASPIRATIONS

ACHIEVEMENTS

habit tracker

(ADD NEW OR GIVE UP OLD)

M	T	W	T	F	S	S
○	○	○	○	○	○	○
○	○	○	○	○	○	○
○	○	○	○	○	○	○
○	○	○	○	○	○	○
○	○	○	○	○	○	○
○	○	○	○	○	○	○
○	○	○	○	○	○	○

THOUGHTS, RANDOM & OTHERWISE

the week of _____

ASPIRATIONS

ACHIEVEMENTS

habit tracker

(ADD NEW OR GIVE UP OLD)

M	T	W	T	F	S	S
○	○	○	○	○	○	○
○	○	○	○	○	○	○
○	○	○	○	○	○	○
○	○	○	○	○	○	○
○	○	○	○	○	○	○
○	○	○	○	○	○	○
○	○	○	○	○	○	○

THOUGHTS, RANDOM & OTHERWISE

the week of _____

ASPIRATIONS

ACHIEVEMENTS

habit tracker

(ADD NEW OR GIVE UP OLD)

M	T	W	T	F	S	S
○	○	○	○	○	○	○
○	○	○	○	○	○	○
○	○	○	○	○	○	○
○	○	○	○	○	○	○
○	○	○	○	○	○	○
○	○	○	○	○	○	○
○	○	○	○	○	○	○

THOUGHTS, RANDOM & OTHERWISE

the week of _____

ASPIRATIONS

ACHIEVEMENTS

habit tracker

(ADD NEW OR GIVE UP OLD)

M	T	W	T	F	S	S
◯	◯	◯	◯	◯	◯	◯
◯	◯	◯	◯	◯	◯	◯
◯	◯	◯	◯	◯	◯	◯
◯	◯	◯	◯	◯	◯	◯
◯	◯	◯	◯	◯	◯	◯
◯	◯	◯	◯	◯	◯	◯
◯	◯	◯	◯	◯	◯	◯

THOUGHTS, RANDOM & OTHERWISE

the month of

HAPPY   "MEH"   TIRED   ANGRY   SAD

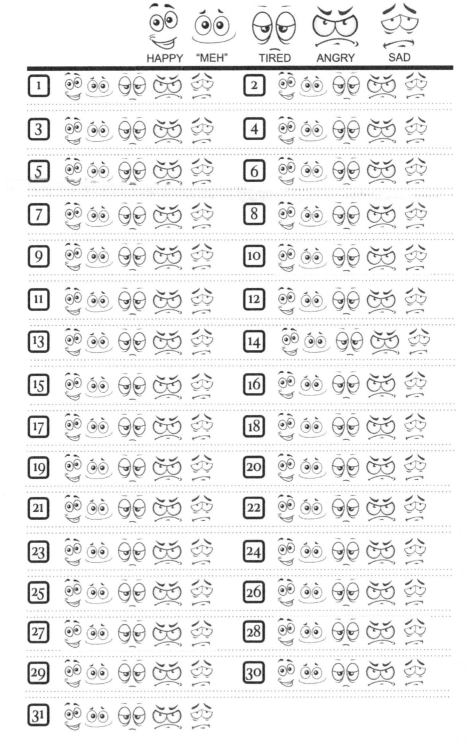

INSPIRATION. MOTIVATION. DETERMINATION.

A PLACE FOR DOODLES, PHOTOS, STICKERS & WHATEVER MOVES YOU

A PLACE FOR DOODLES, PHOTOS, STICKERS & WHATEVER MOVES YOU

WORK IN PROGRESS LOG SHEETS

GAUGE YOUR PROGRESS, BE IT BY SIZE, STRENGTH, WEIGHT, ACTIVITY OR ANY OTHER METRIC THAT LETS YOU KNOW YOU'RE GETTING WHERE YOU WANT TO BE. DESIGN YOUR OWN "BECOMING BETTER" LOG.

what I'm measuring _____

progress bar
(color it in as you succeed)

start [   ] goal!

WORK IN PROGRESS LOG SHEETS

GAUGE YOUR PROGRESS, BE IT BY SIZE, STRENGTH, WEIGHT, ACTIVITY OR ANY OTHER METRIC THAT LETS YOU KNOW YOU'RE GETTING WHERE YOU WANT TO BE. DESIGN YOUR OWN "BECOMING BETTER" LOG.

what I'm measuring _____

progress bar
(color it in as you succeed)

start | | goal!

WORK IN PROGRESS LOG SHEETS

GAUGE YOUR PROGRESS, BE IT BY SIZE, STRENGTH, WEIGHT, ACTIVITY OR ANY OTHER METRIC THAT LETS YOU KNOW YOU'RE GETTING WHERE YOU WANT TO BE. DESIGN YOUR OWN "BECOMING BETTER" LOG.

what I'm measuring _____

progress bar
(color it in as you succeed)

start | | goal!

WORK IN PROGRESS LOG SHEETS

GAUGE YOUR PROGRESS, BE IT BY SIZE, STRENGTH, WEIGHT, ACTIVITY OR ANY OTHER METRIC THAT LETS YOU KNOW YOU'RE GETTING WHERE YOU WANT TO BE. DESIGN YOUR OWN "BECOMING BETTER" LOG.

what I'm measuring _____

progress bar
(color it in as you succeed)

start | | goal!

WORK IN PROGRESS LOG SHEETS

GAUGE YOUR PROGRESS, BE IT BY SIZE, STRENGTH, WEIGHT, ACTIVITY OR ANY OTHER METRIC THAT LETS YOU KNOW YOU'RE GETTING WHERE YOU WANT TO BE. DESIGN YOUR OWN "BECOMING BETTER" LOG.

what I'm measuring _____

progress bar
(color it in as you succeed)

start | | goal!

GAUGE YOUR PROGRESS, BE IT BY SIZE, STRENGTH, WEIGHT, ACTIVITY OR ANY OTHER METRIC THAT LETS YOU KNOW YOU'RE GETTING WHERE YOU WANT TO BE. DESIGN YOUR OWN "BECOMING BETTER" LOG.

what I'm measuring _____

progress bar
(color it in as you succeed)

start [   ] goal!

WORK IN PROGRESS LOG SHEETS

GAUGE YOUR PROGRESS, BE IT BY SIZE, STRENGTH, WEIGHT, ACTIVITY OR ANY OTHER METRIC THAT LETS YOU KNOW YOU'RE GETTING WHERE YOU WANT TO BE. DESIGN YOUR OWN "BECOMING BETTER" LOG.

what I'm measuring _____

progress bar
(color it in as you succeed)

start _____ goal!

WORK IN PROGRESS LOG SHEETS

GAUGE YOUR PROGRESS, BE IT BY SIZE, STRENGTH, WEIGHT, ACTIVITY OR ANY OTHER METRIC THAT LETS YOU KNOW YOU'RE GETTING WHERE YOU WANT TO BE. DESIGN YOUR OWN "BECOMING BETTER" LOG.

what I'm measuring _____

progress bar
(color it in as you succeed)

start | | goal!

WORK IN PROGRESS LOG SHEETS

GAUGE YOUR PROGRESS, BE IT BY SIZE, STRENGTH, WEIGHT, ACTIVITY OR ANY OTHER METRIC THAT LETS YOU KNOW YOU'RE GETTING WHERE YOU WANT TO BE. DESIGN YOUR OWN "BECOMING BETTER" LOG.

what I'm measuring _____

progress bar
(color it in as you succeed)

start | | goal!

AND NOW,
FOR SOMETHING
COMPLETELY GOOFY

KETO
COLORING!

(ANYTHING TO KEEP OUR HANDS & MINDS BUSY, RIGHT?)

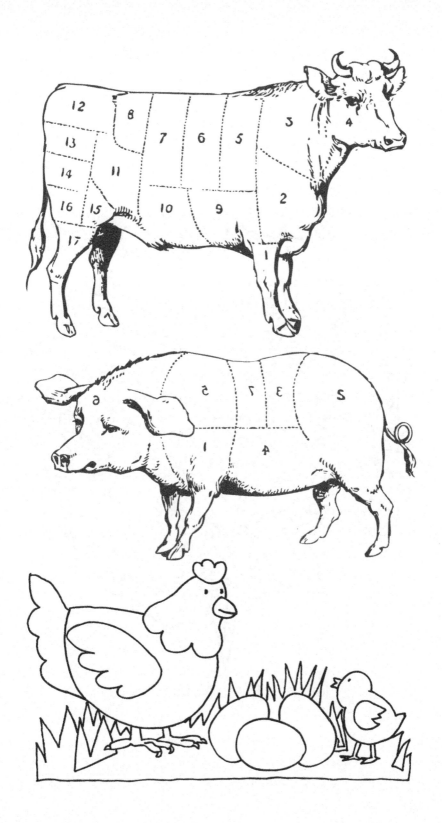

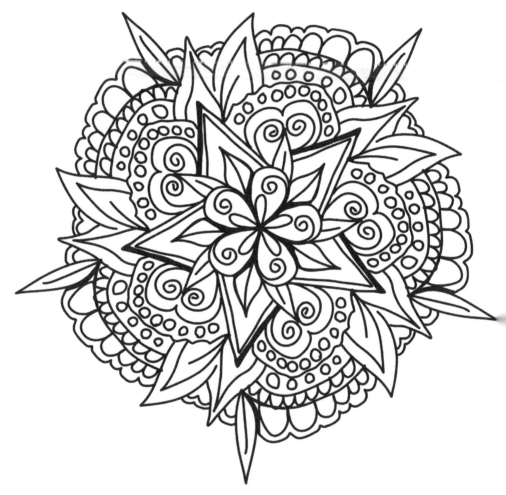

Image by Kaylin Art from Pixabay

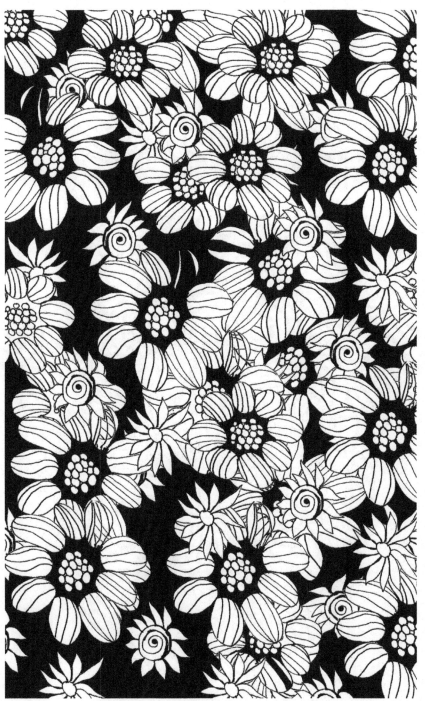

Image by <u>Kaylin Art</u> from <u>Pixabay</u>

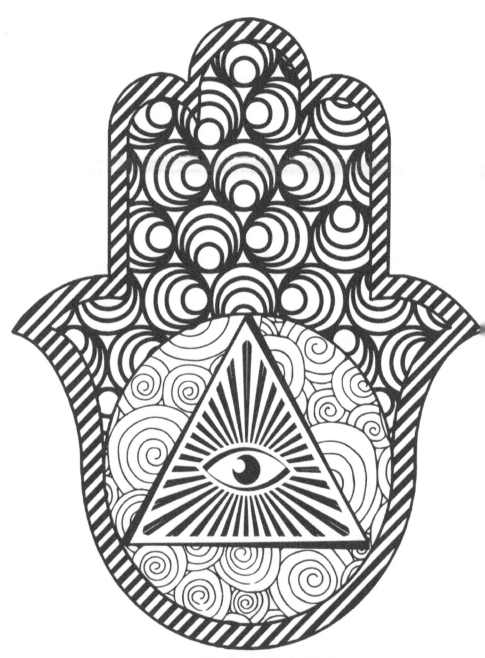

Image by Kaylin Art from Pixabay

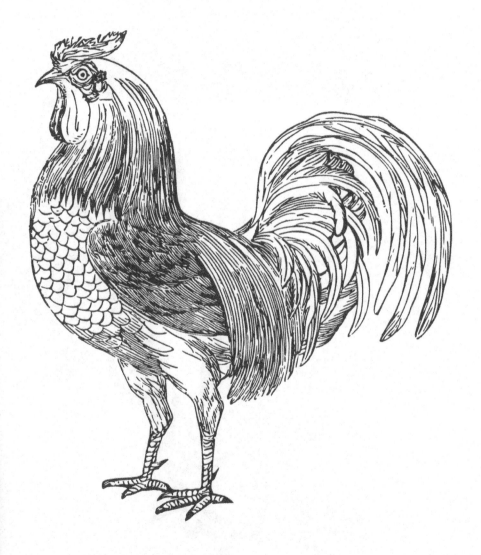

Image by <u>OpenClipart-Vectors</u> from <u>Pixabay</u>

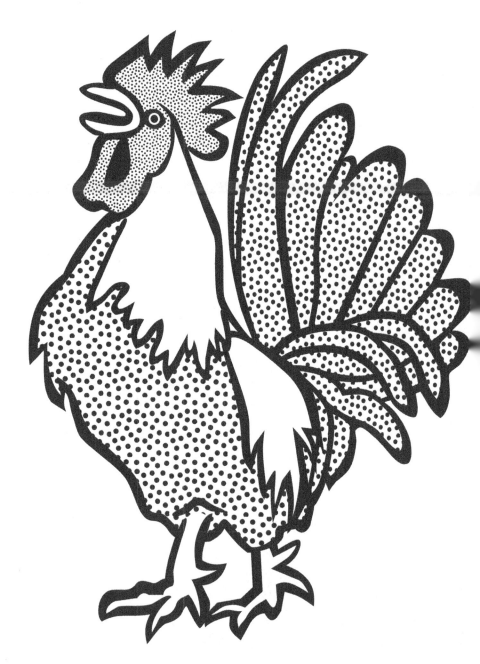

Image by <u>OpenClipart-Vectors</u> from <u>Pixabay</u>

Life is change. Let's embrace that and direct as much of it for ourselves as we can. I hope this little book helped you with that very thing.

Made in the USA
Coppell, TX
01 June 2021